Mediterranean Greens, Sweets & Drinks

An Unmissable Collection of Inspired Recipes for Your Mediterranean Meals

Marta Jackson

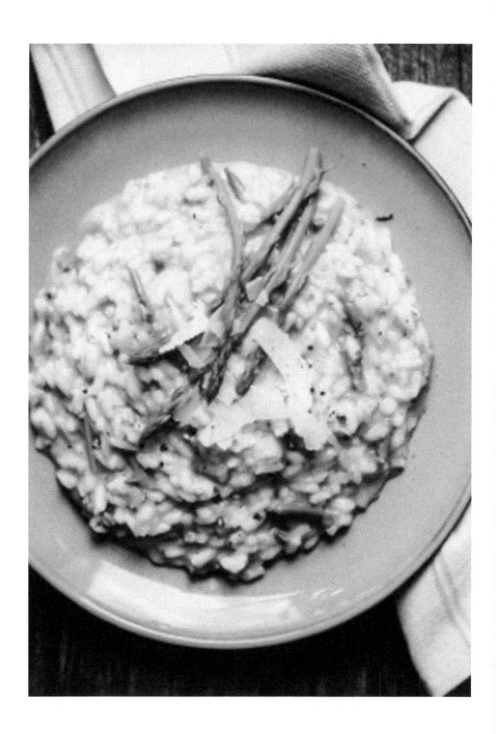

Table of Contents

Pear and ginger pudding

Ingredients

- 1 ripe pear
- Golden syrup
- 1 large free-range egg
- 55g of self-rising flour
- 1 piece of stem ginger in syrup
- 55g of unsalted butter
- 55g of caster sugar
- 1 orange

Directions

- Place 2 teacups upside down on greaseproof paper, draw round them.
- Cut out the circles.
- Grease one side with butter, then grease the inside of the teacups.
- Using a food processor, process the flour together with the sugar, butter, and egg.
- Add the ginger, orange zest, pulse twice.
- Pour a small golden syrup into the base of each cup, top with half the chopped pear each.

- Divide the batter between the two cups, then lightly press a circle of paper on top, butter-side down.
- Let cook in the microwave, full power for 4 minutes.
- Let cool.
- Serve and enjoy with lashings of hot custard.

Berry good pancakes

Ingredients

- 1 handful of blueberries
- 1 cup self-rising flour
- 6 slices of streaky bacon
- 1 teaspoon baking powder
- 1 large free-range egg
- 20g of butter
- 1 cup of milk

Directions

- Crack the eggs, fill the same cup with flour.
- Add to the bowl. Toss in the baking powder.
- Fill the cup with milk, add a tiny pinch of sea salt.
- Whisk till smooth. Cover the bowl in Clingfilm and put to one side.
- Heat a non-stick frying pan, let fry until crisp.
- Put a large frying pan on a medium heat, melt the butter.
- Place the pancake batter into the pan.

- Let cook 2 minutes, until little bubbles rise up to the top. Turnover.
- Dot a handful of blueberries across the half-cooked pancakes.
- Transfer to a plate and cover with foil.
- Add the remaining butter, use all the butter.
- Serve and enjoy with the bacon.

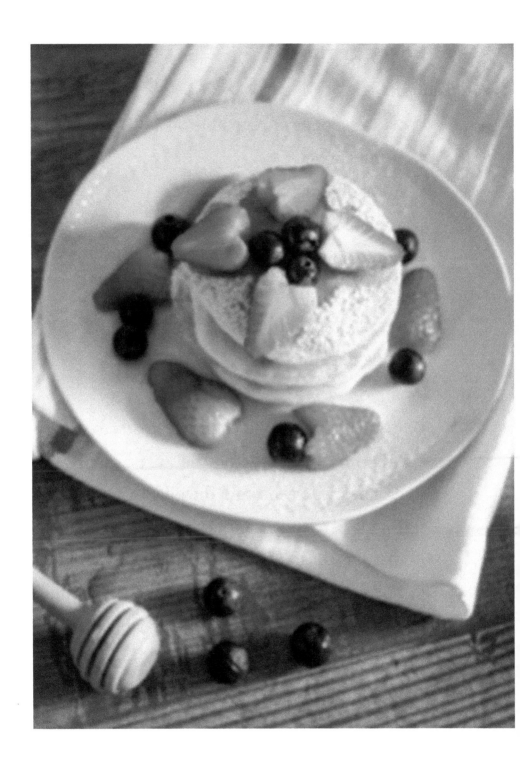

Cranberry granola

Ingredients

- 2 tablespoons of vegetable oil
- Runny honey
- 400g of jumbo rolled oats
- 100g of seeds
- 200g of mixed nuts
- 150g of dried cranberries
- 1 teaspoon of ground cinnamon
- 500g of plain yoghurt

Directions

- Begin by preheating your oven ready to 350°F.
- Mix the nuts with the oats, half the cranberries, seeds, and the oil. Stir.
- Divide between 2 baking sheets, let cook for 25 minutes till golden.
- Mix the yoghurt together with the cinnamon.
- Serve the granola with the yoghurt and a drizzle of honey.
- Enjoy.

Passion fruit cairipinha

Ingredients

- 4 tablespoons of golden caster sugar
- Crushed ice
- 3 limes
- 75ml of cachaça
- 1 ripe passion fruit

Directions

- Begin by cutting the limes into wedges.
- Place the lime wedges except 2 with sugar in a cocktail shaker.
- Muddle briefly to almost dissolve the sugar.
- Add the cachaça, spoon in most of the passion fruit pulp.
- Fill the shaker with crushed ice and shake for 1 minute.
- Pour the cocktail into 2 glasses.
- Use the 2 remaining lime wedges to garnish and the passion fruit pulp.
- Serve and enjoy.

Date, cocoa and pumpkin recipe

Ingredients

- 1 teaspoon of vanilla extract
- 1 orange
- 50g of whole almonds
- 80g of Medjool dates
- 1cm piece of fresh turmeric
- ½ teaspoon of ground cinnamon
- 20g of puffed brown rice
- 1 heaped teaspoon of quality cocoa powder
- 70g of pumpkin seeds
- ½ tablespoon of Manuka honey

Directions

- Expressly, blend 40g pumpkin seeds into a dust in a food processor.
- Add remaining pumpkin seeds with the puffed rice in the processor, almonds, and dates. Blend to chop.
- Add the ground turmeric, with cinnamon, cocoa powder, and a pinch of sea salt.
- Blend again until ground

- Add the vanilla together with the honey and half the orange juice.
- Blend briefly.
- Divide into 24 then roll into balls.
- Throw into the pumpkin seed dust.
- Shake to coat, storing them in the excess dust until needed.
- Serve and enjoy.

Cherry clafoutis

Ingredients

- 60g of sugar
- ½ tablespoon of unsalted butter
- 1 tablespoon of sugar
- ½ teaspoon of vanilla extract
- 300g of cherries
- 300ml of milk
- Icing sugar
- ½ teaspoon of baking powder
- 3 large free-range eggs
- 60g of plain flour

Directions

- Preheat the oven to 360°F.
- Combine plain four together with the baking powder, eggs, sugar, milk, and vanilla extract in a food processor, blend until smooth, keep for 30 minutes.
- Oil a round baking dish with the softened butter.
- Sprinkle over with the sugar.

- Dot the cherries around the base, place in the oven for 5 minutes.
- Remove and pour over the batter until the cherries are just covered.
- Return to the oven let bake for 35 minutes.
- Dust the clafoutis with icing sugar and serve warm.
- Enjoy.

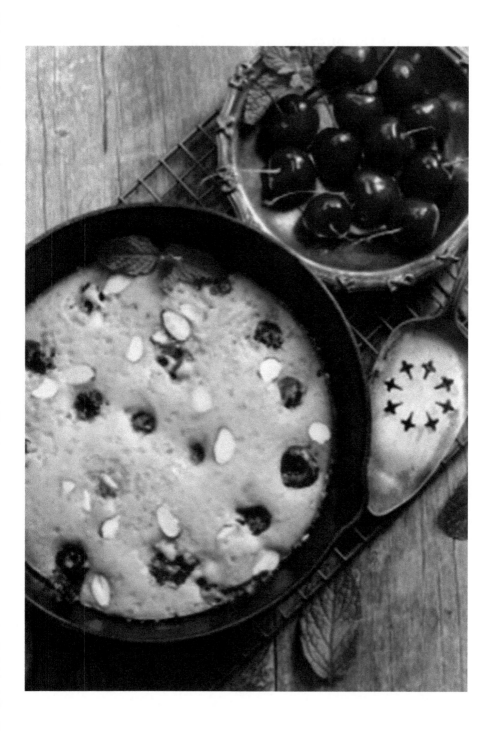

Cranberry Bakewell

Ingredients

- 2 large eggs
- 375g of sweet short crust pastry
- 2 heaped tablespoons of plain flour
- 1 splash calvados
- 1 handful of cranberries, fresh, defrosted
- 250g of unsalted butter
- 1 orange
- 100g of icing sugar
- 375g of cranberries, fresh or defrosted
- 150g of golden caster sugar
- 1-star anise
- 1 orange
- 1/2 teaspoon of ground cinnamon
- 1 vanilla pod
- 300g of ground almonds
- 300g of golden caster sugar

Directions

- Grate the orange zest into a pan.

- Squeeze in the juice, let simmer with the remaining ingredients, stirring occasionally.
- Taste, and adjust accordingly.
- Cool, then remove the star anise.
- Roll out the pastry to line oiled loose-bottomed tart tin.
- Let chill in the fridge for 1 hour.
- Combine vanilla pod, almonds, plain flour, caster sugar, eggs, unsalted butter, and processor, process until smooth.
- Wrap in Clingfilm and chill in the fridge for 30 minutes with pastry.
- Preheat the oven ready to 380°F.
- Line the pastry with greaseproof paper and fill with dried beans.
- Let bake for 10 minutes.
- Remove the beans and paper continue to bake for more 15 minutes.
- Remove.
- Then, spread the pastry with the jam, dollop over the frangipane.

- Sprinkle with the cranberries, scatter with flaked almonds.
- Bake 55 minutes.
- Let tart cool.
- Grate the orange zest into a small bowl.
- Add the icing sugar, squeeze enough orange juice to give a drizzling consistency.
- Serve and enjoy with crème fraiche.

Winter ginger, pear and almond cake

The winter ginger, pear and almond recipe is known for its aromatic ginger flavor with spicy sweet satisfying ingredients. It is an incredible Mediterranean Sea fruit recipe for a perfect breakfast choice.

Ingredients

- 20g of butter
- 220g of ground almonds
- 300g of ginger
- 4 pears
- 200g of butter
- 1 vanilla pod
- 200g of caster sugar
- 550g of caster sugar
- 4 large free-range eggs

Directions

- Preheat the oven ready to 380°F.
- Place the vanilla pod, grated ginger, and pears into a pan.
- Add 400g sugar and water let boil, simmer for briefly.

- Lower the pears into the hot liquid, simmer for 10 minutes.
- Remove the pears from the liquid let cool.
- Line a cake tin with greaseproof paper.
- Combine the remaining 150g sugar and water in a pan over a high heat.
- Simmer for 15 minutes until dark golden brown.
- Stir in the butter until you get a caramel, then pour into cake tin.
- Slices cooled pears, arrange in the warm caramel.
- Mix butter with sugar until smooth.
- Add the eggs one at a time, mix well one after the other.
- Add the almonds and mix to combine.
- Pour the cake mixture over the pears let bake 35 minutes in the heated oven.
- Serve and enjoy.

Summer pudding

Ingredients

- 2 tablespoons of red berry jam
- 150g of sugar
- ½ of an orange
- ½ teaspoon of vanilla paste
- 800g of mixed summer berries
- Olive oil
- 7 large slices of white bread

Directions

- Grease a pudding basin with oil.
- Align with 2 sheets of Clingfilm.
- Place the berries in a large saucepan together with the sugar, orange juice, and vanilla paste.
- Over low heat, let cook for 5 minutes or till the juices start bleeding from the fruit. Let cool.
- Remove the crusts from the bread, spread over the jam.
- Line the basin with 6 of the slices, jam-side up with no gaps.
- Press the bread against the sides.

- Spoon the cooled fruit and pour its juice into the lined basin, reserving some.
- Cover the pudding with the last slice of bread, jam-side down.
- Place a saucer that fits inside the basin on top of the pudding, then place a weight, on top.
- Refrigerate 12 hours to soak the juices.
- Strain the leftover juice through a fine sieve into a small pan.
- Let boil, simmer for 10 minutes.
- Drizzle large slices with the syrup.
- Serve and enjoy with crème fraiche.

Raspberry burnt cream

Ingredients

- 100g of raspberries
- 150ml of double cream
- 4 large free-range egg yolks
- 1 vanilla pod
- 2 tablespoons of golden caster sugar
- 150ml of single cream

Directions

- Preheat the oven to 300°F.
- Add vanilla pod to a pan with the creams over a low heat.
- In a bowl, whisk the egg yolks with sugar.
- Add in the hot cream, whisk frequently to make a custard.
- Strain through a sieve into a jug.
- Boil water.
- Divide the berries between four small ovenproof ramekins, then fill each with the custard.

- Place ramekins in roasting tray, pour in hot water halfway up the sides.
- Let cook in the oven for 20 minutes.
- Remove, let cool, then cover each ramekin with Clingfilm, refrigerate overnight.
- Sprinkle sugar over the custards, burn the top with a blowtorch.
- Allow to stand to let the burnt sugar hardens, then return to the fridge and chill until needed.
- Enjoy.

Citrus poached pears

Ingredients

- Double cream
- 1 lemon
- 2 pears
- 1 stick of cinnamon
- 200g of granulated sugar
- 1 orange

Directions

- Place the peeled zest and juice from the lemon, orange into a saucepan.
- Add the cinnamon together with the sugar, add 500ml of water and bring to the boil, until the sugar dissolves.
- Add the pears into the syrup once the sugar has dissolved.
- Let simmer 12 minutes or until tender.
- Remove and let cool.
- Serve the pears with double cream and or with 4 tablespoons of poaching.
- Enjoy.

Limon cello and fruit salad fro-yo

Ingredients

- 75ml of Limon cello
- 1kg of chopped mixed fruit
- Ice-cream cones
- 250ml of fat-free natural yoghurt
- Runny honey

Directions

- Blend the fruit together with the yoghurt, 2 tablespoons of honey, and the limon cello in a food processor until smooth.
- Taste and adjust accordingly.
- Spoon into a dish and freeze for 2 hours, until frozen.
- Remove and place back into the processor, blend again to break up any ice crystals. Enjoy.

Versatile veggie chili

The versatile veggie chili recipe is quite delicious and a hearty substitution to traditional chili. It features butternut squash, leek and spring onions for a greater flavor coupled with cayenne pepper for a perfect choice of a Mediterranean Sea diet.

Ingredients

- 1 heaped teaspoon ground cumin
- Lime or lemon juice, or vinegar
- Olive oil
- 2 mixed-color peppers
- 2 cloves of garlic
- 1 level teaspoon cayenne pepper
- 2 x 400g of tins of beans
- 1 bunch of fresh coriander
- 2 fresh mixed-color chilies
- 1 onion
- 1 level teaspoon ground cinnamon
- 2 x 400g of tins of quality plum tomatoes
- 500g of sweet potatoes

Directions

- Preheat the oven ready to 400°F.
- Prepare and place chopped potatoes onto a baking tray.
- Sprinkle with a pinch of cayenne, cinnamon, cumin, sea salt and black pepper.
- Drizzle with oil then toss to coat.
- Let roast for 1 hour or until golden.
- Place 2 tablespoons of oil in a large pan over a medium-high heat.
- Add the onion together with peppers, and garlic.
- Let cook for 5 minutes, stirring regularly.
- Add the coriander stalks together with the chilies and spices.
- Cook for more 10 minutes or until softened, stirring occasionally.
- Add the beans, juice and all.
- Tip in the tomatoes, breaking them up with the back of a spoon, stir well.
- Let boil, lower the heat to medium-low for 30 minutes.

- Stir the roasted sweet potato through the chili with most of the coriander leaves,
- Taste and adjust accordingly.
- Add a squeeze of lime or lemon juice or a swig of vinegar.
- Serve and enjoy with yogurt or sour cream.

Classic ratatouille

Ingredients

- 2 red onions
- 4 cloves of garlic
- 2 aborigines
- 3 courgettes
- 3 red or yellow peppers
- 6 ripe tomatoes
- ½ a bunch of fresh basil
- Olive oil
- A few sprigs of fresh thyme
- 1 x 400 g tin of quality plum tomatoes
- 1 tablespoon of balsamic vinegar
- ½ of a lemon

Directions

- Start by heating 2 tablespoons of oil in a large casserole pan over a medium heat.
- Add the chopped aubergines together with the courgettes and peppers.
- Let fry for 5 minutes, spoon the cooked vegetables into a large bowl.

- Add the onion, garlic, basil stalks, and thyme leaves with another drizzle of oil to the pan.
- Let fry for 15 minutes or until golden.
- Return the cooked veggie to the pan.
- Stir in the fresh and tinned tomatoes together with the balsamic and a pinch of sea salt and black pepper.
- Cover and let simmer over a low heat for 35 minutes.
- Tear in the basil leaves, grate in the lemon zest.
- Taste and adjust seasoning accordingly.
- Serve and enjoy with steamed rice.

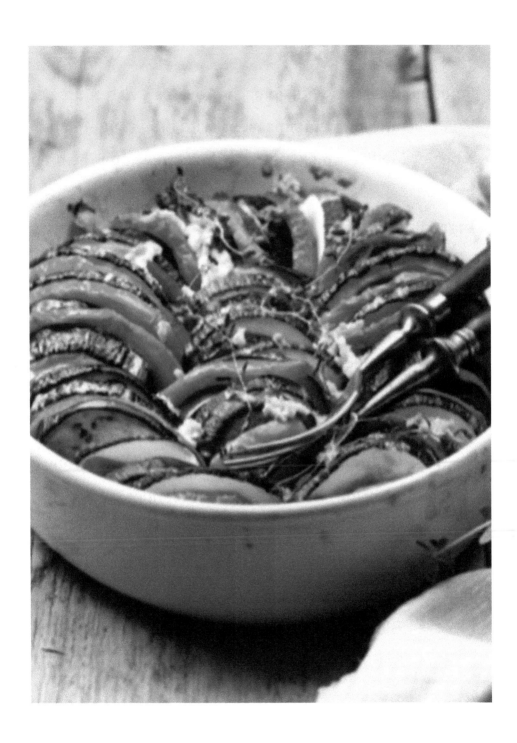

Carrot spinach juice

Combining carrots with spinach provides a rich source of iron, calcium, and vitamins along with other mineral. It is a tastier Mediterranean juice with a simple step-by-step method.

Ingredients

- 6 medium size carrots
- 1 large bunch of spinach
- Celery stalk
- ½ of lemon
- 1 ½ cups of water

Directions

- Combine the carrots together with the celery stalk and all the water in a blender.
- Blend to puree.
- Then, add the spinach and juice of lemon, (squeeze).
- Blend briefly, then, strain.
- Serve and enjoy.

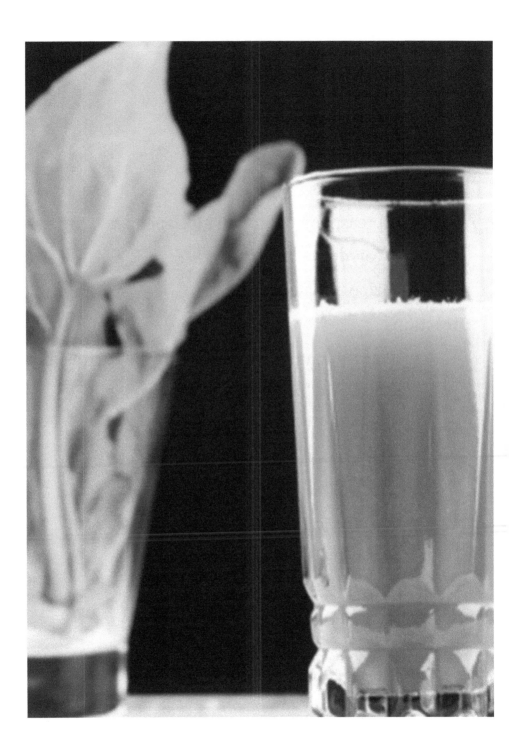

Fresh tomato juice

Ingredients

- Celery stalks
- Salt
- 2 ice cubes
- ¼ teaspoon of ground black pepper
- 2 carrots
- 6 ripe tomatoes

Directions

- Place tomatoes together with the carrots and celery in a blender.
- Blend until smooth.
- Then, add salt with black pepper to season, mix well.
- Add the ice cubes in serving glasses.
- Serve and enjoy.

Aubergine parmigiana

This a great meal recipe originating from the parts of northern Italy making a perfect Mediterranean Sea diet with variety of vegetables. It can be served perfectly with roasted fish.

Ingredients

- 1 bunch of fresh basil
- A few sprigs of fresh oregano
- 3 large firm aubergines
- 2 handfuls of dried breadcrumbs
- 150g of buffalo mozzarella
- Olive oil
- ½ a bulb of spring garlic
- 1 heaped teaspoon dried oregano
- 2 x 400g tins of quality plum tomatoes
- Wine vinegar
- 1 onion
- 3 large handfuls of parmesan cheese

Directions

- Preheat a griddle barbecue ready.

- Place a large pan on a medium heat with olive oil.
- Add the onion together with the garlic and dried oregano.
- Let cook for 10 minutes.
- Add the tomato flesh to onion pan, stir well, cover and let simmer 15 minutes over low heat.
- Grill the aubergines on both sides until lightly charred.
- Season the tomato sauce with sea salt, black pepper and a tiny swig of wine vinegar.
- Pick in the basil.
- Spoon a layer of tomato sauce into a baking dish.
- Add a scattering of Parmesan, then single layer of aubergines.
- Repeat these layers until all the ingredients are used.
- Toss chopped oregano with breadcrumbs and some olive oil.
- Sprinkle on top of the Parmesan.
- Tear over the mozzarella.

- Let bake 30 minutes.
- Serve and enjoy.

Bubble and squeak

Ingredients

- 600g of leftover cooked vegetables.
- 600g of leftover roast potatoes
- olive oil
- leftover vac-packed shell nuts
- 25g of unsalted butter
- 4 sprigs of fresh woody herbs

Directions

- Place a non-stick frying pan on a medium heat with little olive oil and butter.
- Pick in the fresh herb leaves, let crisp up briefly.
- Add the potatoes, vegetables, and any leftover shell nuts.
- Season with sea salt and black pepper.
- Let cook for 4 minutes or until golden crust forms on the bottom.
- Using a fish slice, fold crispy bits back into the mash.

- Let crisp up again, then repeat the process for 20 minutes.
- Taste and adjust the seasoning accordingly.
- Serve and enjoy with fried eggs and or lemon-dressed watercress.

Speedy quiche tray bake

Ingredients

- 6 medium free-range eggs
- 1 x 250g pack of ready-rolled filo pastry
- 55g of mature Cheddar cheese
- 1 large courgette
- 1 bunch of spring onions
- Olive oil
- 300g of broccoli

Directions

- Start by preheating the oven ready to 350°F.
- Then, grease a large roasting tray with bit of olive oil.
- Crack the eggs into a bowl and beat well.
- Layer the filo sheets into the tray, laying one sheet horizontally, and the next vertically, repeating as you layer.
- Bush with bit of egg between each sheet.
- Add a final brush to the last layer and scrunch up any excess pastry.

- Add slice spring onions, cheddar cheese, courgette, and broccoli to the bowl.
- Season with sea salt and black pepper, mix.
- Pour the mixture into the prepared pastry case, spreading out.
- Sprinkle the remaining cheese over the top.
- Let cook for 35 minutes, until the pastry is golden.
- Serve and enjoy.

Roasted parsnips

This recipe is infused with the acidity of the vinegar that strikes through the entire recipe with bay and honey.

Ingredients

- 4 fresh bay leaves
- 2 tablespoons of runny honey
- 1.5kg of medium parsnips
- 1 tablespoon of white or red wine vinegar
- 50g of unsalted butter

Ingredients

- Firstly, preheat your oven ready to 350°F.
- Blanch whole in a large pan of boiling salted water for 5 minutes.
- Drain off the water and steam dry.
- Tip into a large roasting tray.
- Dot over the butter and a pinch of sea salt and black pepper, toss to coat.
- Organize in a single layer, let roast for at least 1 hour.
- Remove from oven, quickly scatter over the bay leaves.

- Drizzle with the vinegar and honey, toss together.
- Continue to roast for 10 minutes or until golden.
- Serve and enjoy.

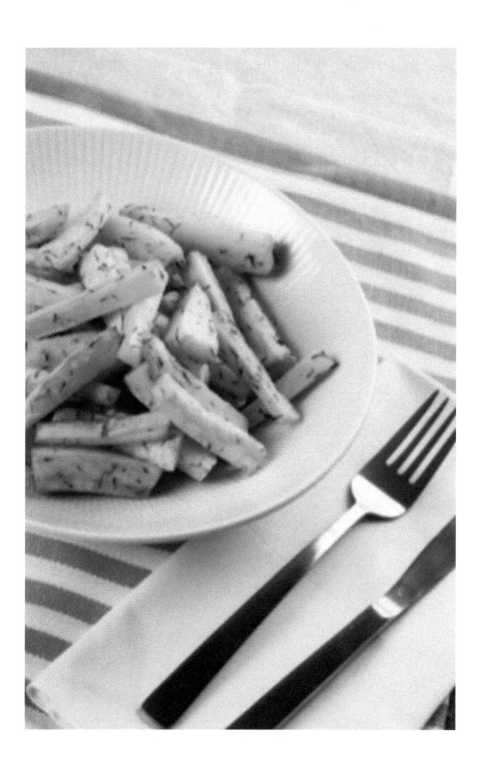

Veggie Bolognese sauce

Ingredients

- 250g of alliums
- 1 liter tomato base sauce
- 12g of garlic
- 1 tablespoon of dried mixed herbs
- 1 veggie stock cube
- 750g of Mediterranean veggies
- 25ml of olive oil
- 250g of lentils

Directions

- Place a large pan to hold all the ingredients on a medium heat with the olive oil.
- Add the alliums together with the garlic.
- Let cook for 20 minutes.
- Add the chopped Mediterranean vegetables with the herbs.
- Let cook for 15 minutes or until the vegetables are golden.
- Crush the vegetables.

- Add the lentils with the tomato base sauce, boil.
- Add water and stock cube stir well.
- Boil, lower the heat, let simmer for 40 minutes.
- Season with sea salt and black pepper.
- Serve and enjoy.

Veggie korma

Ingredients

- 2 x 400g tins of chickpeas
- 500g of alliums
- lemon juice
- 175g of plain yoghurt
- 350ml of white base sauce
- 30ml of olive oil
- 2 tablespoons of curry powder
- 2 teaspoons of smoked paprika
- 1kg of mixed vegetables
- 750ml of curry base sauce

Directions

- Place all the ingredients in large a pan over medium heat with the oil.
- Add the alliums together with the curry powder and smoked paprika.
- Cook until the alliums are golden in 20 minutes stirring frequently.
- Add chopped vegetables apart form leafy greens, to the pan, cover let cook briefly.

- Pour in the curry and white sauces with the chickpeas and water.
- Bring to the boil, lower the heat let simmer for 35 minutes.
- Add the reserved leafy vegetables.
- Boil again, let cook until the curry has reduced.
- Stir in the yoghurt until warmed through.
- Season with lemon juice, salt and black pepper.
- Serve and enjoy.

Freezer raid springtime risotto

Ingredients

- 300g of mixed frozen green vegetables
- 1 liter of vegetable stock
- Extra virgin olive oil
- 1 onion
- 1 stick of celery
- 60g of freshly grated parmesan cheese
- 1 lemon
- Olive oil
- 2 knobs of unsalted butter
- 300g of risotto rice
- 125ml of white wine

Directions

- Simmer the stock in a pan over a low heat.
- Place 1 tablespoon of olive oil together with knob of butter, onion, and celery into a pan over low heat.
- Season lightly with sea salt and black pepper.
- Cook for 10 minutes, stirring occasionally, until the vegetables are soft.

- Increase the heat to medium.
- Add the rice and stir for 2 minutes, pour in the wine and stir to absorb.
- Add hot stock, stir until fully absorbed, then add more.
- Cook for 18 minutes, adding more stock every minute, stirring regularly.
- Stir in the frozen veggies to cook through 5 minutes to rice cook time.
- Stir in the remaining butter and the Parmesan, season accordingly when heat is off.
- Drizzle with extra virgin olive oil, squeeze in bit of lemon juice per portion.
- Enjoy.

Glazed carrots

Ingredients

- 50g of unsalted butter
- 2 fresh bay leaves
- 1 tablespoon of dripping
- 2 clementine
- 2 tablespoons of runny honey
- 1kg of small mixed-color carrots
- 6 cloves of garlic
- 8 sprigs of fresh thyme

Directions

- Melt the butter in a large frying pan over a medium heat.
- Add crushed garlic to the pan, turn frequently.
- Sprinkle in the thyme sprigs, clementine juice and honey, bay, and a splash of water.
- Add the carrots, sprinkle with sea salt and black pepper, shake to coat.
- Cover, lower heat to medium-low let cook for 15 minutes.
- Serve and enjoy.

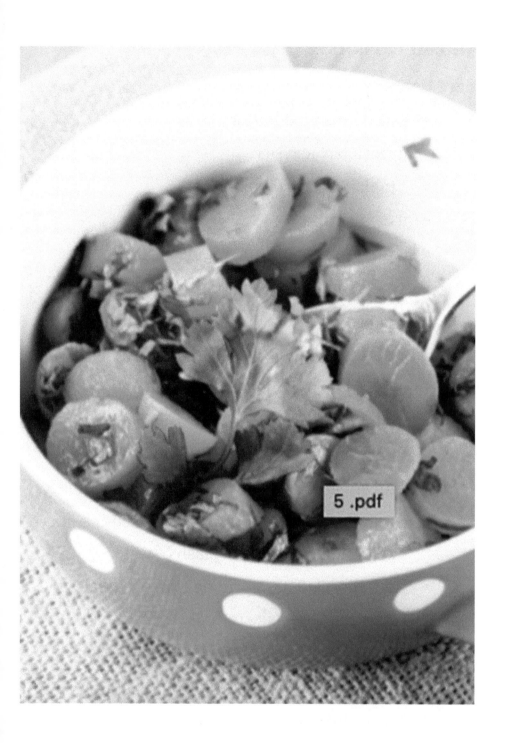

5 .pdf

Brussels sprouts

The Brussels sprouts are insanely delicious with apple cubes, Worcestershire and sausages for a great Mediterranean Sea diet.

Ingredients

- 1 sweet eating apple
- 1 tablespoon of Worcestershire sauce
- 2 higher-welfare Cumberland sausages
- 1 onion
- 800g of Brussels sprouts
- ½ a bunch of fresh sage
- 20g of unsalted butter

Directions

- Cook the Brussels in a large pan of boiling salted water for 5 minutes.
- Drain any excess water, let steam dry.
- Melt butter in a large frying pan on a medium-low heat.
- Add half the sage leaves and let cook for 3 minutes, transfer into a small bowl.

- Place the pan back on the heat, add the sausage to the pan.
- Cook for 5 minutes, until golden.
- Add the onion with the chopped sage let cook for 5 minutes over medium heat, stirring occasionally.
- Add sliced apples with sprouts, Worcestershire sauce and toss.
- Serve and enjoy with scatter sage leaves on top.

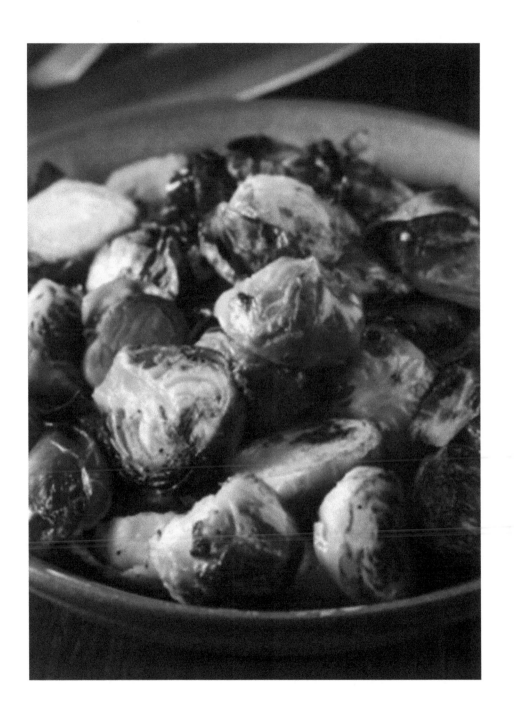

Classic apple crumble

The classic apple crumble is a homely Mediterranean fruit recipe, simple and delicious for breakfast.

Ingredients

- 100g of plain flour
- 150g golden caster sugar
- 1 lemon
- 50g of unsalted butter
- 1.5kg of mixed apples

Directions

- Preheat your oven to 400°F.
- Peel and core the apples.
- Place in a saucepan over medium heat with sugar and some gratings of lemon zest.
- Cook for 5 minutes with the lid on.
- Lower the heat and let cool.
- Place butter in a mixing bowl with flour.
- Rub together with your fingertips until it resembles breadcrumbs and add the remaining sugar.
- Transfer the apples to a baking dish.

- Sprinkle over the crumble topping.
- Bake for 25 to 30 minutes.
- Serve and enjoy with vanilla.

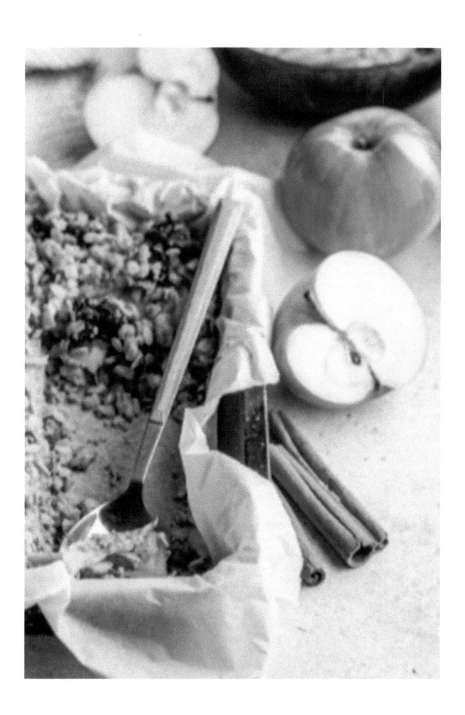

Following these procedures for making scones can yield better of this meal than a store bought scones. They are quiet simple and ease to make, tasty when still fresh from the oven.

Ingredients

- Orange juice, for soaking
- Jersey clotted cream, good-quality jam or lemon curd
- 4 tablespoons of milk
- 500g of self-rising flour
- 2 level teaspoons of baking powder
- 150g of dried fruit
- 2 heaped teaspoons of golden caster sugar
- 150g of cold unsalted butter
- 2 large free-range eggs

Directions

- Place dried fruit into a bowl.
- Add orange juice to cover let stay for hours.
- Preheat your oven to 400°F.

- Combine the butter, flour, sugar, baking powder, and a good pinch of sea salt ina mixing bowl.
- Break and rub the butter with your fingers.
- Make a well in the middle of the dough.
- Add eggs and milk.
- Stir up with a spatula.
- Drain soaked fruit, add to the mixture.
- Add a tiny splash of milk.
- Sprinkle over some flour, cover the bowl with Clingfilm, keep in the fridge briefly.
- Roll the dough out on a lightly floured surface until it's about 3cm thick.
- Cut out circles from the dough and place them upside down on a baking sheet.
- Brush the top of each scone with the extra milk.
- Bake in the oven for 15 minutes.
- Serve and enjoy with clotted cream.

Apple and walnut risotto with gorgonzola

Ingredients

- Freshly ground black pepper
- 1 basic risotto recipe
- 1 handful of walnuts
- 75g of soft goat's cheese, crumbled
- 700ml of organic vegetable
- Extra virgin olive oil
- 50g of butter
- 1 small handful of Parmesan cheese
- 1 small bunch of fresh marjoram
- Sea salt
- 175g of gorgonzola cheese, diced
- 2 crunchy eating apples

Directions

- Place a large saucepan on a medium to high heat.
- Pour in half the stock, then the risotto base.
- Bring to the boil, stirring all the time, lower the heat, let simmer until almost all the stock has been absorbed.

- Add the rest of the stock, bit by bit until the rice is cooked.
- Turn off the heat, beat in the butter together with the Parmesan, goat's cheese, chopped apple, gorgonzola, and marjoram.
- Taste, and adjust the seasoning.
- Let the risotto rest briefly, covered with a lid.
- Heat the walnuts in a pan.
- Serve and enjoy with a sprinkle of the walnuts and drizzle with a little extra virgin olive oil.

Apple and cranberry sauce

Ingredients

- 1 stick of cinnamon
- 500g of cranberries
- 150g of golden caster sugar
- 2 bramley apples

Directions

- Place all the ingredients in a wide saucepan with a splash of water.
- Place the pan on heat and bring to the boil.
- Simmer gently until the cranberries have burst and the apple are soft.
- Boil down until the mixture thickens slightly.
- Remove, let cool.
- Serve and enjoy.

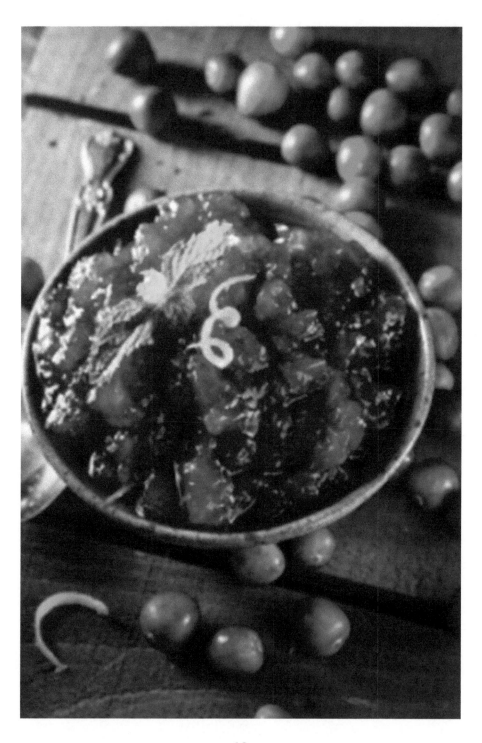

Summer crunch salad with walnuts and gorgonzola

Ingredients

- 200g of gorgonzola cheese
- 1 lemon
- Extra virgin olive oil
- 2 bulbs fennel, thinly sliced
- 3 large handfuls fresh peas
- 2 handfuls walnut halves
- 2 small red apples

Directions

- Squeeze the lemon through your fingers into a mixing bowl, make sure to catch any pips.
- Add 3 times as much olive oil to the lemon juice.
- Season with sea salt and freshly ground black pepper. Whisk.
- Core and thinly slice each apple.
- Then, toss with the fennel and walnuts in the dressing.
- Divide between smaller dishes.

- Crumble the Gorgonzola over the top of each.
- Serve and enjoy.

Apple and celeriac soup

Ingredients

- A few sage leaves
- A few sprigs of thyme
- 4 tablespoons of olive oil
- 4 apples
- 2 liters of vegetable stock
- 2 onions
- Toasted hazelnuts
- 200ml of crème fraiche
- 1 celery stalk
- 1 celeriac

Directions

- Heat half of the olive oil in a large pan.
- Cook slice onions with chopped celery over a medium heat for 10 minutes, or until soft.
- Chop the celeriac, core and quarter the apples, add to the pan with thyme leaves, let cook for 3 minutes.

- Add the stock, season, over low heat let simmer for 30 minutes until the celeriac is tender.
- Remove from heat, blend until smooth. Stir in half the crème fraiche.
- Heat the remaining oil in a pan and fry the sage leaves until crispy.
- Spoon the soup into bowls, topping with the remaining crème fraiche.
- Drizzle with extra virgin olive oil and sprinkle with the crispy sage leaves and hazelnuts.
- Enjoy.

Waldorf salad

Ingredients

- 2 crisp eating apples
- 150g of grapes
- 6 sprigs of fresh tarragon
- 250ml of fat-free natural yoghurt
- 2 sticks of celery
- 1 lemon
- Olive oil
- 1 teaspoon of English mustard
- 60g of shelled walnuts
- 1 cos, or Romaine lettuce

Directions

- Preheat your oven ready to 350°F.
- Place the grapes on a baking tray, finely grate over the zest from ½ the lemon, and drizzle with a little oil.
- Season with sea salt and black pepper.
- Then, place in the hot oven for 15 minutes.
- Add the walnuts, let roast for more 10 minutes.

- Place the mustard with yoghurt into a dish, whisk.
- Add the chopped tarragon leaves and squeeze in the lemon juice, mix, then season to taste.
- Place chopped celery and sliced apples, lettuce, grapes into a large bowl.
- Drizzle over the yoghurt dressing and toss well.
- Place onto a platter, roughly chop and sprinkle over the walnuts.
- Serve and enjoy.

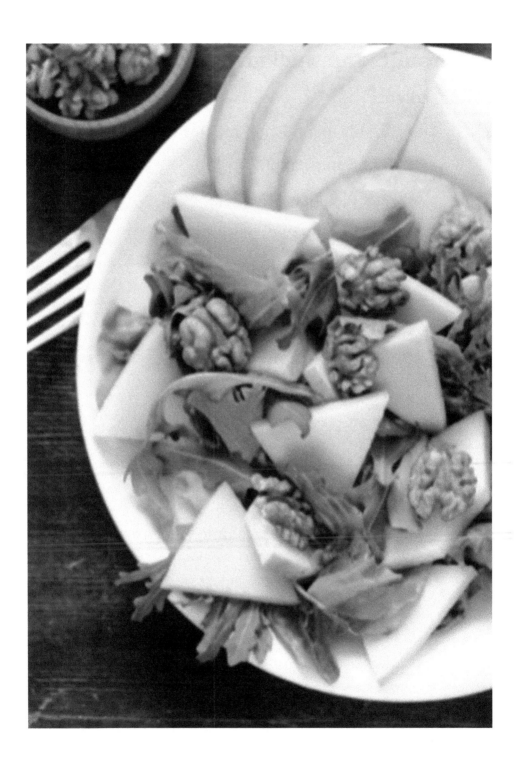

Parsnips and shell nut tart tatin

Ingredients

- 1 tablespoon Dijon mustard
- ½ bramley apple
- 20g of goose fat
- ½ tablespoon of balsamic vinegar
- 50g of unsalted butter
- ½ tablespoon of runny honey
- 2 parsnips
- 100g of ready-to-cook shell nuts
- 7 sprigs of thyme
- 320g if ready-rolled puff pastry
- ½ tablespoon of dark brown sugar
- 3 shallots
- 1 tablespoon of balsamic vinegar
- 200g of shallots
- 50g of dates
- ½ tablespoon of olive oil

Directions

- Preheat the oven to 400°F.

- Heat olive oil in a medium pan over a medium-low heat.
- Add the shallots, let cook for 5 minutes, until tender.
- Stir in the mustard together with the balsamic, dates, honey, sugar, and water.
- Season, and lower the heat, let cook for 15 minutes, stirring occasionally,
- Remove, let cool.
- Heat the goose fat and butter in an ovenproof frying pan over a medium-low heat.
- Then, add the parsnips together with the shallots, cut-side down, let cook until it begins to caramelize.
- Add the shell nuts with thyme sprigs, season, let cook for 5 minutes.
- Remove from the heat and top with half of the shallot compote.
- Roll out the pastry and trim it so it's slightly bigger than the pan.
- Remove the pan from the heat and roll the pastry over the top.

- Let bake for 30 minutes, until the pastry is golden.
- Simmer the apple with water in a small pan over a medium heat for 10 minutes.
- Season and stir in the balsamic.
- Serve and enjoy hot with the apple balsamic sauce on the side.

Cheat's cranberry sauce

Ingredients

- 1 x 250g jar of cranberry sauce
- 1 eating apple
- 1 cinnamon stick
- 1 fresh bay leaf
- 1 knob of unsalted butter

Directions

- Place a pan on a medium heat with the butter, cinnamon, and bay.
- Let cook briefly for 40 seconds, or until the cinnamon starts to catch and burn.
- Stir in the cubes of apple and a swig of water, shake to coat in the butter.
- Leave to soften for a couple of minutes.
- Pour in the cranberry sauce, let warm through.
- Serve and enjoy.

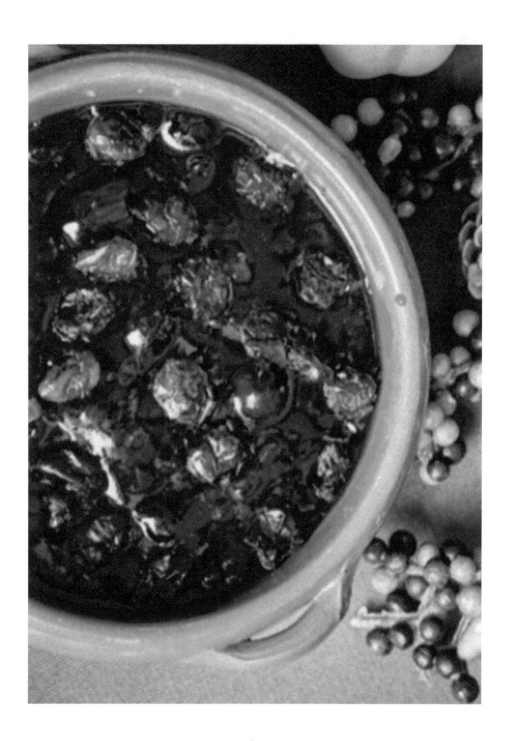

Grapefruit, carrots, and apple juice

Ingredients

- ½ of a grapefruit
- 1 apple
- 3 medium carrots

Directions

- Peel the grapefruit, and quarter the apple.
- Push the grapefruit with the carrots and apple through a juicer, straight into a glass.
- Stir well.
- Enjoy.

Blue cheese and apple burger

Ingredients

- Mustard
- 750g of minced chuck steak
- 6 burger buns
- 1 soft round lettuce
- Olive oil
- 120g of blue cheese
- 1 punnet of cress
- 2 Brae burn

Directions

- Divide the mince into 4 portions and work each ball in your hands for a few minutes to melt the fat.
- Mold them into a relatively smooth, round patty. Make sure they are bigger than the burns.
- Place them on a tray cover with Clingfilm, let chill in the fridge.
- Preheat your grill to high.

- Place a large non-stick frying pan over a medium heat and add a drizzle of oil to the pan.
- Let fry the burgers for 4 minutes on each side.
- Seasoning the patties with black pepper as you cook them.
- Halve and toast the buns under the grill, then line them up on a board ready to go.
- When the burgers are cooked, top each with the blue cheese, place under the grill for a couple of minutes until oozy.
- Now build your burgers. First layer the salad leaves and apple onto the buns, then drizzle of mustard.
- Place the burgers on, topping with the cress.
- Enjoy your delicious.

Fried cox apples with cinnamon sugar

Ingredients

- 1 teaspoon of ground cinnamon
- 250g of unsalted butter
- 4 tablespoons of caster sugar
- 4 Cox orange pippin apple
- Apple juice
- 1 lemon

Directions

- Begin by clarifying the butter by boiling in a small pan.
- Strain into a container through a sieve lined with a coffee filter.
- Peel, core and slice each apple into 8, then sprinkle over a little lemon juice to prevent the slices from browning.
- Heat some clarified butter in a non-stick frying pan.
- Add the apple pieces in one layer.
- Let cook until the undersides are nicely tanned.

- Combine the sugar together with the cinnamon, turn over the apple slices and sprinkle with the cinnamon sugar.
- Lift the apples into a dish.
- Pour a splash of the apple juice in the pan.
- Serve and enjoy.

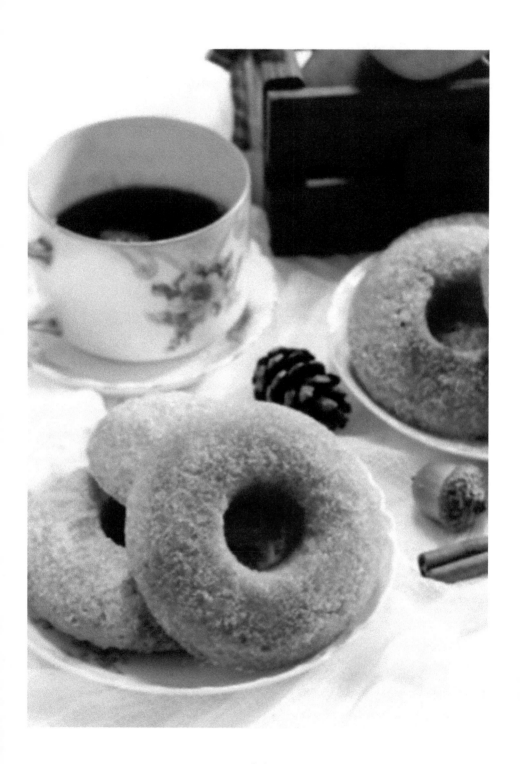

Celery juice

The celery juice is an excellent source of dietary fiber significant for calorie weight loss plans. More so, it is a tasty and a refreshing with a rejuvenating property for a daily diet. A person cannot love Mediterranean diet without loving this juice.

Ingredients

- 2 celery sticks
- 1 apple
- ¼ od ginger
- ¼ of lime or lemon

Directions

- Clean all the ingredients.
- Place all ingredients except lime or lemon in a blender or juicer
- Blend thoroughly.
- Squeeze lemon over the juice
- Serve and enjoy chilled.

Apple ginger juice

Ingredients

- 3 apples
- ½ piece of ginger
- ½ lemon
- ½ cup of water

Directions

- Clean and chop the apples.
- Combine apple, ginger and the water in the juicer.
- Squeeze the lemon in.
- Blend until smooth puree.
- Strain and sieve the juice.
- Serve and enjoy immediately.

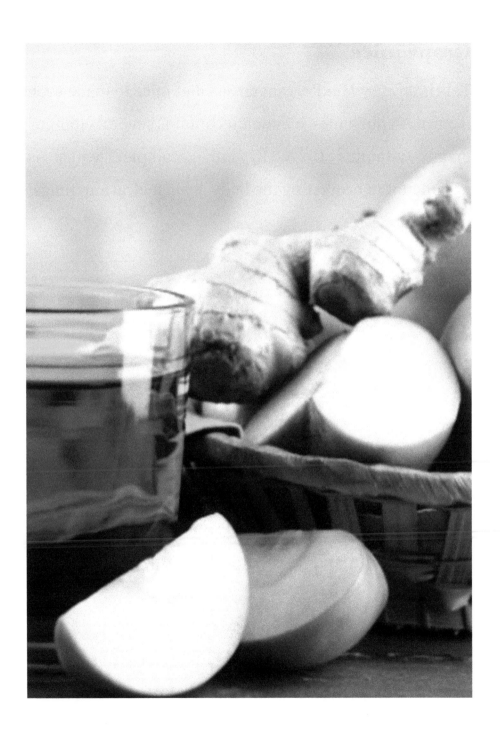

Grape juice

This is an easy Mediterranean Sea diet juice to make even if one does not have a blender. It contains several vitamins mainly vitamins C, A, K, and B-complex which is paramount in protecting the body against viral and fungal infections.

Ingredients

- 2 cups of sweet ripe black grapes
- ½ lemon
- 1 cup of water
- 8 ice cubes.

Directions

- Clean and place the grapes in a blender.
- Add the water.
- Run the blender until smooth.
- Strain and sieve, and then squeeze the lemon over.
- Adjust the thickness with more water.
- Serve and enjoy chilled or at room temperature.

Strawberry raspberry smoothie

Ingredients

- ½ cup of raspberries
- ½ cup of frozen strawberries
- ½ of banana
- ¼ cup of plain yogurt
- ½ of almond milk
- ½ teaspoon of chia seeds
- ½ tablespoon of honey

Directions

- Pour almond milk together with the yogurt in a blender.
- Then, add the raspberries, banana, chia seeds, honey, and strawberries.
- Run the blender until smooth.
- Serve and enjoy.

17. Pomegranate juice

Ingredients

- 1 cup of fresh pomegranate seeds
- ½ cup of water

Directions

- Cut and remove the pomegranate crown, and make shallow cuts on the skin, make sure to deseed.
- Place 1 cup of pomegranate seeds in a blender.
- Add the water.
- Pulse to break the seeds a little.
- Strain and sieve.
- Serve and enjoy.

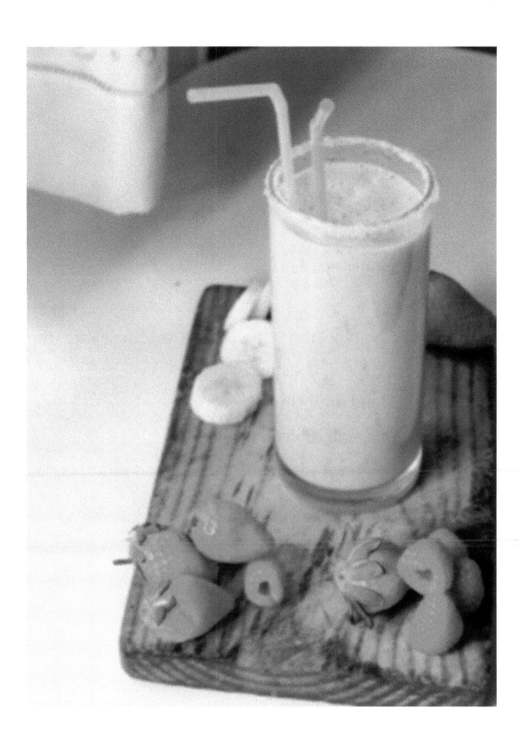

Strawberry juice

Ingredients

- 2 cups of ripe strawberries
- 1 tablespoon of honey
- 1 cup of cold water
- 2 ice cubes
- 1 halves strawberry

Directions

- Combine the strawberries together with the honey in a blender.
- Blend until smooth puree.
- Add water, blend briefly.
- Serve with ice cubes and halved strawberries on the rim of the serving glasses.

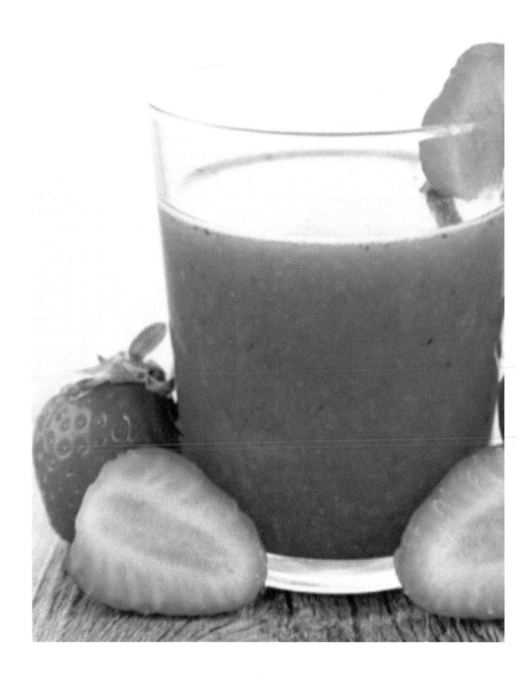

Orange pineapple juice

This Mediterranean Sea diet juice is largely an orange juice with little taste of pineapple. The orange pineapple juice is a tasty and delicious recipe, but its health and nutrition benefits supersedes its taste.

Ingredients

- 4 oranges
- 1 pinch of ground black pepper
- 1 cup of water
- Salt
- 2 cups of chopped ripe pineapples
- Honey

Directions

- Cut and halve the oranges.
- Squeeze the juice with a juicer.
- Place pineapples, honey, sugar, salt, and ground black pepper in a blender.
- Blend until smooth puree.
- Strain, then add the orange juice, mix.
- Serve and enjoy.

Pineapple juice

Ingredients

- 1/2 ripe pineapple
- ½ cup of water
- 6 ice cubes
- Honey

Directions

- place chopped pineapple and water in a blender.
- Process until smooth puree without chunks.
- Strain properly.
- Add ice cubes and stir well.
- Taste and adjust sweetness accordingly.
- Serve and enjoy.

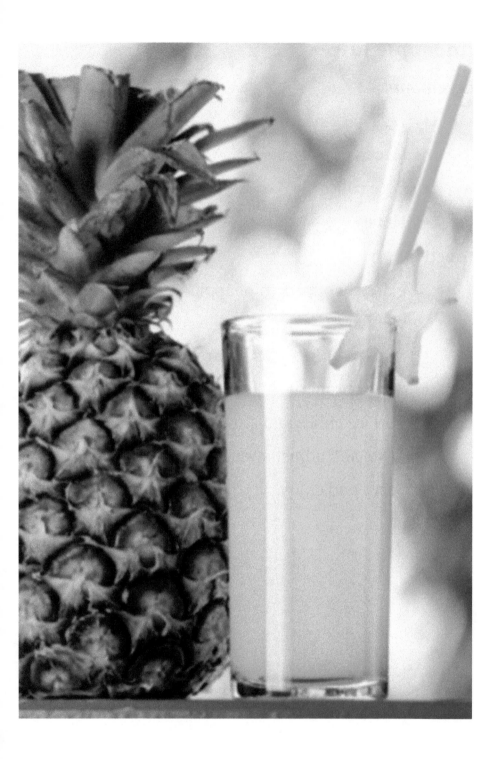

Orange juice

Ingredients

- 3 fresh oranges
- Ice cubes

Directions

- Clean and roll the oranges on a flat surface to soften.
- Cut crosswise and place in a juicer.
- Squeeze the juice.
- Strain to trap the seeds.
- Serve with ice cubes, garnishing with the orange wheel.
- Enjoy.

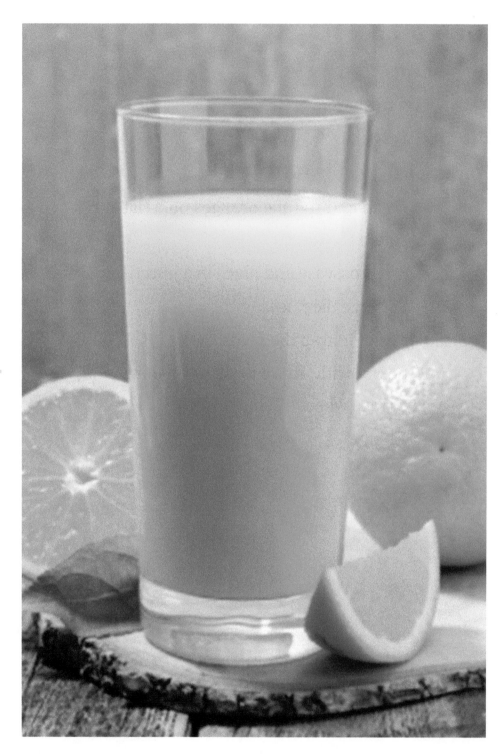

Apple orange juice

Ingredients

- 1 sweet apple
- 2 oranges
- ¾ cup of water
- 2 teaspoons of honey

Directions

- Chop and prepare the oranges, remove the skin and seeds.
- Place in a juicer, and squeeze out the juice.
- Add water, chopped apples, and juice from the oranges in a blender.
- Blend until smooth puree.
- Strain.
- Then, add honey, mix.
- Serve and enjoy.

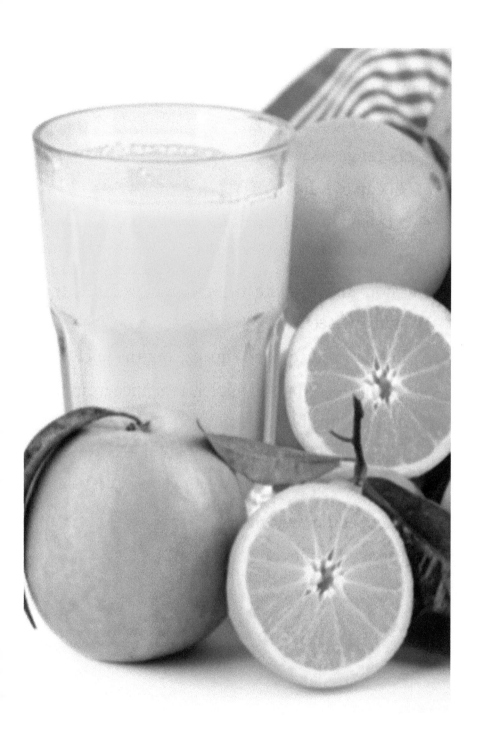

Banana orange juice

Ingredients

- 2 oranges
- 6 ice cubes
- 1 medium banana

Directions

- In a juicer, squeeze the lemon juice.
- Transfer to a blender.
- Then, add the chopped banana with ice cubes.
- Blend until smooth and puree.
- Serve and enjoy.

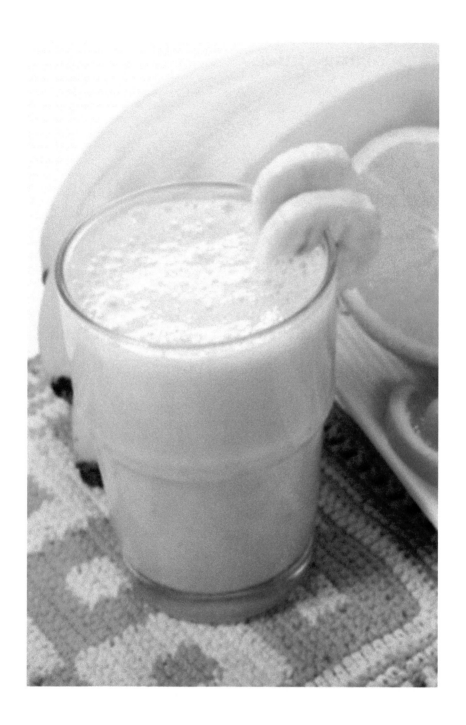

Fresh spinach juice

Ingredients

- 2 cups of chopped spinach
- 1 stalk of celery
- Juice from ½ lemon
- ¾ cup of water
- 1 apple

Ingredients

- Place the apple, celery, and water in a blender.
- Then, add the spinach and lemon juice.
- Blend until smooth without chunks.
- Strain.
- Serve and enjoy chilled or at room temperature.

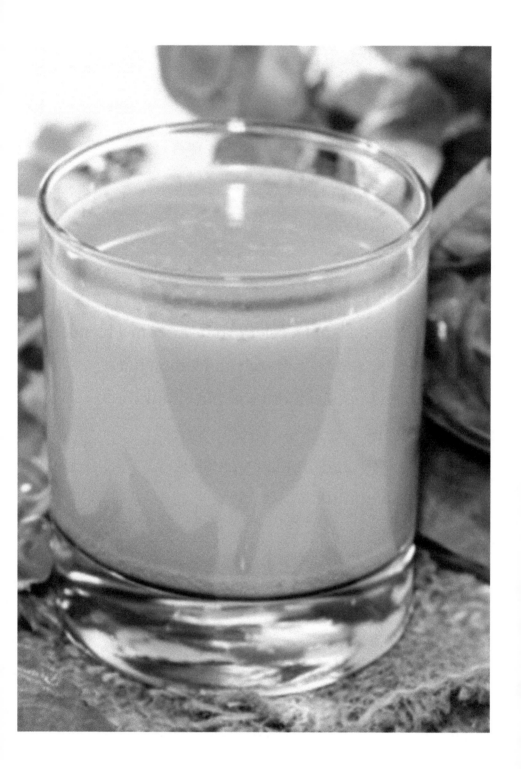

Kiwi juice

Ingredients

- 1 celery stalk
- Apple
- Kiwifruit

Directions

- Clean and slice the apple and kiwifruit.
- Place the slices of apples and kiwifruit with celery stalk in a juicer.
- Process using an omega masticating juicer.
- Serve and enjoy.

Papaya juice

Ingredients

- 2 teaspoons of lemon juice
- ½ medium size papaya
- ½ cup of fresh pineapple juice
- 2 teaspoons of honey
- 1/8 teaspoon of black pepper powder
- Salt
- Water

Directions

- Place the papaya, pineapple juice, black pepper powder, lemon juice, honey, salt, and water in a blender.
- Blend until smooth puree.
- Check and adjust the consistency with pineapple juice, blend briefly.
- Taste, and adjust the sweetness with honey or lemon juice, making it tangy.
- Serve and enjoy chilled.

Sweetheart slaw with passion fruit dressing

Ingredients

- 1 carrot
- 1 sweetheart cabbage
- 1 large orange
- 3 large spears of asparagus
- 2 tablespoons of cold-pressed extra virgin olive oil
- 1 tablespoon of poppy seeds
- 3 spring onions
- 3 ripe passionfruit
- 2 sticks of celery
- 1 large green eating apple

Directions

- Grate the orange zest into a bowl and squeeze in all the juice.
- Halve the passion fruit and scrape in the pulp, then add the olive oil, mix together.
- Place shredded cabbage, asparagus, spring onions, apple, and carrot into a large bowl.

- Pour over the dressing, mix, season to taste.
- Serve and enjoy immediately.